CW00400616

30-DAY GUIDED
WEIGHT LOSS
PROGRAM

Optimum Combination of
Intermittent Fasting | Dieting
Running | Skipping

Rajat Gajbhiye

ISBN-13: 9798838606501

Cover design by: Adhishri Rays

CONTENTS

INTRODUCTION

This book is going to be short and sweet. I will stick to only those things which are necessary to understand this weight loss program. It takes a lot of effort for months to get the weight loss result you want. Suppose you want to lose 30 pounds and decide to lose 5 pounds per month, then it will take 6 months to get that result. What if I told you that you could get the same result in a month? Yes, it is possible. Don't worry; there won't be any side effects to losing that much weight so fast. Some people or books will claim that losing weight that fast is not healthy. Of course, it is healthy. If you think it's not healthy, then you are totally underestimating the capabilities of your body.

If you lose 30 pounds in a month, you will save 5 months of your life. You will be really happy to see "New You" in the mirror every day. Your confidence will be boosted, and people will praise you and ask you how you achieved it.

But have you ever realized how much effort you need to put in to get that result? If your answer is – A LOT, then that's the wrong answer. The correct answer is 10 TIMES A LOT (10 x A LOT). It will be much harder than you are thinking right now.

If you say you'll work on losing weight but not too hard, I'm sorry to say you've chosen the wrong book, my friend. You will be wasting your time if you read another page of this book. Because let me make myself very clear; you will not achieve that good result in such a short period if you don't work your ass off. And if you have prepared yourself mentally to work really hard to shed that extra fat that has been lying with you for so long, then I heartily welcome you to this most amazing "30-Day Guided Weight Loss Program."

HOW IT ALL STARTED?

When I was a trainer in the gym, I met a gym client. His name was Mr. Anil Sharma, age 38. He was 172 cm tall and weighed 246 pounds. He was a software engineer. Despite having a hectic office schedule, he used to find time for the gym every day. For one year, he used to come to the gym consistently, but there was no significant change in his body. When his 1-year gym membership expired, he did not renew it for the next year. I remember it very clearly. Wednesday was the last day of his gym. In the locker room, he was packing his gym bag. We were the only two in that room. I asked him casually, "Mr. Anil, I heard that you are not renewing the gym membership; what happened?" The answer he gave me led to the birth of this 30-Day Guided Weight Loss Program.

There were only two of us in that room, and maybe so Mr. Anil could speak his heart out to me. He said, "Rajat, I was quite fit when I graduated from engineering college, but gradually life's responsibilities started burdening me."

"It was not that I did not know at all that my

weight was increasing slowly; of course I knew. But I always thought that I should first settle down in life and then pay attention to my body. But I was unaware of the fact that a person never settles down. I was searching for a job after college, then a home after job, then marriage, then children, and life goes on and you don't even realize that 14 to 15 years have gone by."

"A year ago, I was looking at the family album and I realized that I was fat in every photo for the last 12 years. I had completely forgotten that I had once promised myself that I would pay attention to my body. What happened to that promise? To fulfill that promise, I joined this gym. I have been coming to the gym consistently for a year. Do you see any changes? To be honest, I don't have the patience anymore. I was fat before. I am still fat and will probably remain fat in all the photos to come till my death."

Mr. Anil had become quite demotivated. I felt from my heart that this man was genuine and should be helped. I asked him, "Mr. Anil, will you be happy if you see visible results within a month?"

"Visible results?" he asked. "What do you mean by that?"

"We will aim to lose around 20 pounds," I said.

"20 pounds in a month!" he exclaimed. "I've lost less than 10 pounds by going to the gym for an entire year, and if I can lose even 5 pounds in one month, I'll be overjoyed."

"Great."

"Should I extend the gym membership?" he asked.

"No, it won't be necessary," I said. "We will do this weight loss program under the open sky."

"That sounds great; when can we start?" "I'm feeling very excited," he exclaimed.

His face was lighting up like a little child. I was really happy that I had shown a glimmer of hope to a sad and hopeless person. To be honest, I had no idea how this weight loss program was going to work, because I had never done anything like that before.

"I will contact you next week after planning your weight loss program." I said.

"Okay, I look forward to your call," he said. "Thank you, have a great day, bye-bye."

"Bye, see you soon, Mr. Anil."

For the next 7 days, I sat with pen and paper and, by applying all my life's knowledge and experience; I prepared a 30-day weight loss program for Mr. Anil. I knew that this program would work but did not know how much. Because till now it was only on paper, the time had come to try it in practice.

I called Mr. Anil and asked him to meet me exactly at 6 a.m. the next day. We met the next morning; I explained the program to him and said that the success of this program would be determined by his dedication. The more he follows it with dedication, the more success he will get. He agreed to everything I said, and we started our 30-day weight loss program.

We started this program on the 12th of March and it ended exactly 30 days later, i.e., on the 10th of April. The results we got were quite shocking. Although we had set a target of 20 pounds, in reality, it seemed to me that around 10 to 12 pounds would be lost. But both of us were quite surprised by the result we got. Mr. Anil weighed 228 pounds when he started this program, and if I tell you the exact figures, on the 30th day, his weight was 196 pounds. He had lost 32 pounds in 30 days.

In the last 14 years, whenever he used to stand on the weighing machine, its needle would always go above 200. Today, after so many years, when Mr. Anil saw that needle coming down below 200, he became a bit emotional. Although he tried his best to control his emotions, his eyes reflected the truth inside.

We discussed my fees before starting the program, and I stated that if we do not achieve the desired results, I will not charge you any fees, but if we do, you may pay me Rs. 5000 as my fee. I was financially very weak at that time, so Rs. 5000 meant a lot to me. Mr. Anil was so happy with this result that he doubled my fees and handed me a check for Rs. 10,000.

His wife, children, and friends were all surprised by Mr. Anil's transformation. I asked Mr. Anil to come to the gym once and meet his friends. He came, and the gym staff and everyone else were quite surprised to see him. Everyone started asking him how he did this. Inviting Mr. Anil to the gym had two benefits: his confidence increased further and I got two more clients from his praise.

Mr. Anil wanted to go from 196 pounds to

150 pounds now. We also achieved this 46-pounds journey in the next few months. We made the necessary changes in the program and got the result of 150 pounds. Today, Mr. Anil is 146 to 148 pounds. He does not let his weight go above 150 pounds.

Once he achieved his dream weight, I gave him the program on how to maintain it and how to adopt a healthy lifestyle. Mr. Anil was my first client. Even though his result was quite shocking, there were some shortcomings in that 30-day weight loss program.

As my clients grew from word-of-mouth, I gradually worked on making that program the best 30-Day Guided Weight Loss Program in the world. Today I have a full-fledged program. I use the same program for every client. At the moment when I'm writing this book, I'm working with my 526th client.

When I used the same 30-Day Guided Weight Loss Program on my first 100 clients and everyone got the best results, I thought I would convert this program into a book. I wanted to reach the maximum number of people who needed to lose weight quickly. But after Mr. Anil's result, I started having a lot of clients. I could not find time for this book. When I had completed 500 clients, I started taking on very selective clients. I only accepted clients who were in desperate need. I kept getting extra time and went on writing this book.

If I tell you the exact figures, out of my 525 clients, the lowest achievement in the 30-Day Guided Weight Loss Program is 12.7 pounds and the highest is 42.5 pounds. Of course, every person's body is different, every person's efforts are different, and every client's goal is different, so the results are different. When I averaged out the weight loss results of all the clients, I got the digit of 26 pounds. This result was good. I was happy that my program changed the lives of many people. When happiness comes into people's lives because of you, it gives you inner happiness. I want to increase that happiness. I want to spread this program to the whole world. I hope this program makes your life better.

WHAT IS 30-DAY GUIDED WEIGHT LOSS PROGRAM?

Nowadays, people want quick results in everything. Many people get it too. But when it comes to losing weight, people say that you have not become so fat in a day. For years, you have been eating a lot of food and becoming fat. When it has taken so long to become fat, then how do you expect that your weight will reduce immediately? That too will take years.

But the good news for you is that even though your weight has increased gradually, it can also be reduced quickly. As the title of the book suggests, we will lose weight in the next 30 days. But how are we going to do it? That's the main question. The 30 day weight loss program consists of the following key factors:

1. Running
2. Skipping
3. Intermittent Fasting
4. Diet And Nutrition

As far as exercise is concerned, we will be doing only two exercises; running and skipping. As we progress through the program, we will gradually increase the intensity of the above four factors.

Every day of this 30 day guided weight loss program has been planned for you to do what you need to do. According to everyday guidance, you should follow everything that is written in the program. Avoid doing anything less or more because the success of this program lies in its particular format.

In today's world, everyone has some knowledge about exercise, diet, intermittent fasting, and most of the things related to health and fitness. Everyone knows the importance of all these, but still only 5% to 10% of people can achieve good fitness, and this is because they are not aware of the process of using all these methods in the best possible way. In this book, we will discuss some of these methods in their optimum form, so that we can get the maximum result in the minimum time.

We will learn about all the four factors in detail and how to use them efficiently for our benefit. You can also go through this program as a challenge, because every day you will be given a new task. And the intensity of the task will increase day by day.

Below is an example of what a typical challenge day will look like.

DAY 15

RUNNING
Depart (D) - 1.7 Miles
Arrive (A) - 1.7 Miles
Total Running = 3.4 Miles

SKIPPING - 300 Skips

DIETING - 2 MEALS - 1600 Calories

INTERMITTENT FASTING
Fasting Window - 16 hours
Eating Window - 8 hours

DATE- _____

☐   I have completed my running challenge for today.
☐   I have completed my skipping challenge for today.
☐   I have followed my diet and intermittent fasting for today.

I am feeling great and have endless energy. I am mentally and physically ready for my 16th day challenge. Let's lose this damn weight faster.

HOW TO START THE PROGRAM?

A] Photographs:

Take photographs of your current body shape. We want to see the visible difference, and for that, photographs will be required. You have to click photos in the following manner.

1. Front, Back, and Side Angles: Full Length (Top to Bottom).
2. Medium length (just below the waist): Front angle

B] Avoid Measuring:

Do not trap yourself in the measurement of your body parts. We are here to make a visible difference. No one will come up to you with a tape, measure your tummy, and exclaim, "Oh, congratulations! It's amazing that you've lost one inch."

We want people to say, "You look different; what are you doing?" "How many pounds have you lost?" And that will be your real achievement. The only thing you have to measure is your current weight. Stand on the weighing scale and take photos of the digits. We will need it for sure.

C] **Things we need:**

Before we start the program we need to have the following things,

1. Running shoes
2. Skipping rope
3. Smart fitness watch or mobile fitness app
4. Protein supplement
5. Multivitamin capsule

I assume that most of you have these top 3 things and do not need to spend your money on them. As far as protein supplements and multivitamin tablets are concerned, if you purchase them in the quantity required for a month, it will be great. Because as the program progresses, we will reduce the number of calories. It's very difficult to get the proper amount of nutrients only through food and with such a small amount of calorie intake. If you can manage this expense for the next 30 days, it will be great for your healthy weight loss program.

RUNNING

Running is mankind's very first exercise. How? When humans hunted animals, they had to run to catch them. Running for 30 minutes burns more calories than doing weight training in the gym for the same time.

As cheese is the main ingredient in the recipe for pizza, similarly, running is the main element of our program. Are you tempted by the word pizza now? I know. It happened to me when I was writing. Anyway, let's get back to the topic. So, in this 30-Day Guided Weight Loss Program, you have to run every day.

Running alone has far more benefits than any other exercise. Studies show that runners live longer than those who don't. Running strengthens your heart and bones. It boosts your mood. There are many reasons why you should start running and make it a daily habit. Let's focus on what type of running you need to do for this program.

You have to run on the road or trail under the open sky. Avoid running on the treadmill. The running time and distance will gradually increase every day.

Running is best done in the morning. If you live in the city, there will be less pollution and fewer vehicles on the road. If you live in the countryside, you will get fresh air in the morning. We usually don't get enough vitamin D. But if you run in the morning, your bones will benefit from that too.

We will use 2 terms while running every day.

1. Depart (D)-Running away from home
2. Arrive (A) – Running towards Home

Suppose your running target for today is 4 miles. Then you have to start running from your home towards your destination for 2 miles; that will be your Depart (D) distance, and come back home for another 2 miles; that will be your Arrive (A) distance.

How should I run?
Stretching:

It is necessary to do a bit of stretching every day before running. You can do head-to-toe full-body stretching for 4 to 5 minutes. It will help you release any tension in your muscles, and you will not feel any kind of stiffness while running.

My few clients preferred walking over running. And their common question was, "Can I do brisk walking instead of running?" The answer to that was, "No."

It doesn't matter how fast you walk, this program demands running. You can run as slowly as you want, but you have to run. Any type of walking is not beneficial for this program.

As you progress through this program, your running distance will increase. Let's say your running goal is 3 miles. If you get tired after running for 1.5 miles, you can walk for 300 to 500 meters comfortably by taking some rest. Once you are reenergized, you can start running again.

The distance covered in this program is more important than the speed at which you run. To complete your running goal is the most crucial factor. Running slow, running at a medium speed, or running at a faster speed doesn't really matter. I leave the speed to you. You can run at the speed you find comfortable running. You can also take some rest when you are tired. You can also relax by walking for a few meters. Whatever it is, you have to cover the distance. This should be your main objective.

You can wear a fitness smartwatch or install a fitness app on your smartphone to keep track of how many miles you run. Remember that you have to use them only for distance measurements; you do not have to get into all those figures of how many calories you have burned. You can also use a waist pouch or small backpack for running. Several items can be kept in this pouch, such as a water bottle, skipping rope, mobile phone, etc., but when you run, the waist pouch, backpack, and stuff you keep in it should not jump. It should be well tied to your body and you should not have any problems with it while running.

We will start by running 0.5 miles on the first day

and gradually increase the distance as we progress. On the 30th day, you will run for 10 miles. Even though we increase the distance gradually over 30 days, it is true that running is a challenging task, especially for those who have never run before or have never considered it as an exercise before. We will need a good amount of motivation, dedication, and sacrifice for that.

The 10 Miles Marathon is the most effective way to stay motivated for 30 days. There are many marathons being held in your city. You can choose any 10-mile marathon event after a month and register for it in advance. If your city does not host a marathon, there are many virtual marathons. This can be done by running 10 miles in your city or village on that particular day and sending them a photo or screenshot confirming you have completed the race in that amount of time. After that, they will send you the medal by courier. That will be your reward.

Your motto is to prepare yourself for that event a month from now. You have to run that 10-mile race with everybody else and finish it with pride. This goal of preparing yourself for a 10-mile marathon will keep you motivated throughout this 30-Day Guided Weight Loss Program.

SKIPPING

S kipping is another effective form of exercise to target your fat loss. It has all the benefits of running. So we will be skipping after running.

After you complete your running target for the day, take a rest for 5 to 10 minutes depending on the miles you ran that day, and start jumping rope. The number of skips will increase as the number of running miles increases. Let's say you have to hit 100 skips. Then you can divide it into 3 sets of 40-30-30 or whatever you are comfortable with. During running, we learned that speed does not make a difference, but distance does. In the same way, in skipping, it does not matter how many sets you take to complete your 100 skips. What matters is, have you completed your goal for today or not?

Now, what should be the speed of skipping? I will leave that to you. Do it at the speed that you like. You just have to complete the target for the day.

Who shouldn't run or jump rope?

Both activities involve increased ground reaction forces. Thus, both activities may be difficult for people with lower leg injuries at the hips, knees, or ankles. When you weigh more than 300 pounds and can't jump rope, you should run slower. If you have an injury in your lower body, then you should try swimming, cycling, and walking. These are forms of exercise where there is less ground reaction force as compared to running and skipping.

Running and jumping rope are both excellent forms of exercise. They're cheap and require minimal equipment. Also, they both burn a significant number of calories in a short amount of time. This can help reduce your body fat percentage and improve your body composition.

INTERMITTENT FASTING

In the last two decades, the practice of intermittent fasting has become very popular, and its popularity is increasing day by day. We get to see the practice of fasting from ancient India. In ancient India, saints used to fast. When they sat to meditate, they managed to get so much control over their mind and body that they could survive for months without food or water. Even today, science has not been able to figure out how any human being can survive without water for so many days. It is obvious that due to not eating or drinking anything for so many days, the saint had become so thin that even their bones were visible.

The most common intermittent fasting method is 16:8, which requires you to fast for 16 hours and eat for the remaining 8 hours of a 24-hour day. Let me explain to you the basic fundamentals behind intermittent fasting in easy language.

Suppose you had your first meal at 12 o'clock in the afternoon. Then you could eat from 12 p.m. to 8 p.m. You have to finish eating the last meal before 8 p.m. And then, from 8 p.m. to 12 p.m. the next day, you do not have to consume anything, not even a single calorie. If you want, you can have black filtered coffee in the morning, which contains 0 calories. You can also drink water, or you can take any drink available in your location that has 0 calories.

Let's throw some light on what happens in your body. When you wake up in the morning in fasting mode, you start feeling hungry a few hours after getting up, and in general, you quench that hunger by having breakfast. But in intermittent fasting, we do not have breakfast. When you are hungry and you eat breakfast, your body uses that food to burn energy. However, what if your body is asking for food but you don't give it any?

Your body needs energy to work and it is not getting it from food, so your body will begin taking energy from stored fat. And that is the whole purpose of intermittent fasting. We want your body to burn stored fat for energy. Suppose you eat something by accident, then your body will stop taking energy from fat and start taking energy from the newly acquired food.

Suppose you have taken the last meal of your day at 6 p.m. Now your body will start digesting what you ate that day. Suppose by 6 a.m. the next morning, you had spent 90% of the energy you had from the food you ate the previous day and only 10% was left. Now you have put on your running shoes and left to run. In total, you ran 3 miles and did 100 skips. Let's say you ran 1 mile and your remaining 10% energy is exhausted. Now your body will start taking energy from the stored fat to run the remaining 2 miles and do 100 skips. It's the only way to burn your fat fast. And if you put calories in between these periods, then your body fat will remain the same. Because then you are not letting your stored fat supply you with energy to do work. So, in simple terms, in intermittent fasting, you have to use the stored fat in your body.

The most common intermittent fasting occurs in the ratio of 16:8, i.e., a fasting window of 16 hours and an eating window of 8 hours. You have to manage these 16 hours and 8 hours according to your job schedule, meetings, travel schedule, etc. There is no hard and fast rule that 16 and 8 hours should be from this time to this time. But there should be a minimum fast of 16 hours. This rule is strict. The intensity of intermittent fasting, i.e. the amount of time spent fasting, will increase as the program progresses. Fasting and eating window will be in the ratio of 16:8, 18:6, 20:4, 23:1.

The intermittent fasting schedule of most of my clients was as follows.

A] Ratio - 16:8
11 a.m. to 7 p.m. - 8-hour eating window
7 p.m. to 11 a.m. - 16-hour fasting window
B] Ratio - 18:6
11 a.m. to 5 p.m. - 6-hour eating window
5 p.m. to 11 a.m. - 18-hour fasting window
C] Ratio - 20:4

11 a.m. to 3 p.m. - 4-hour eating window

3 p.m. to 11 a.m. - 20-hour fasting window

D] Ratio - 23:1

11 a.m. to 12 p.m. - 1-hour eating window

12 p.m. to 11 a.m. - 23-hour fasting window

When you start intermittent fasting, at the beginning and even when you fast for a long time, say 20 or 23 hours, you will feel a little dizzy. But don't worry, that's OK. Our body is not accustomed to this routine, but it is very much capable of it. For a few days, you will feel it, and then it will be normal.

The schedule of all my clients was only in the morning, and it is necessary for you to know the reason behind that. According to the schedule above, morning time is the last 20% to 30% of the fasting window. You've almost used up all of the calories from the previous day's food by then, and if we exercise now, we'll be directly targeting the fat. Morning exercise gives us the best results. After waking up in the morning, the most important thing would be to run and skip. Once you have done that, then you will be free for the whole day to do any work you want.

If you keep the schedule of running and skipping for the evening, then the chances are very high that some other important and urgent work might come up. Our minds are constantly looking for reasons to put off or postpone difficult tasks. And if we don't exercise even for a single day, then our entire routine of 30 days will be disturbed.

Guys, this program is only for 30 days, and if you want the best results, then you have to make it your priority.

DIET AND NUTRITION

In a 16:8 intermittent fast, let's see how we should divide our meals and what we should eat exactly during the 8-hour eating window.

This eating window will be for 8 hours at the start of the program. However, as we progress, this eating window will get shorter and our calorie intake will also decrease. So, in such a situation, we need to take care of our nutrition. In intermittent fasting, people sometimes eat very high-calorie foods in the eating window, like pizza, burgers, and cokes, because the fasting window compensates for those high calories. But to achieve our goal in this 30-Day Weight Loss Program, we will follow a healthy diet and avoid high-calorie foods.

You have to include the following things in your eating window.

1. Vegetables
2. Fruits
3. Grains
4. Nuts and dried fruits.
5. Protein
6. Multivitamins

Now you can get the four things mentioned above through food. However, it is a bit difficult to get your body the required daily amount of protein and all the multivitamins through food, especially when your calorie intake is low. And if you are a vegetarian or vegan, it becomes more difficult to meet the daily requirement for protein. That's why we'll add protein supplements and multivitamin tablets to the program; so that our bodies can obtain the nutrients they need even when calorie intake is low. Initially, we will consume 3 meals per day, and then it will come down to 1 meal per day. When the proportion of meals is low, our body cannot get essential nutrients from food, and for that, we need to add supplements.

If you want to purchase the most reliable protein supplements and multivitamins, then you can compare different companies at labdoor.com. They do genuine lab tests of these products and can tell you the proportion of ingredients and vital data. You can buy the finest supplements available at your location. For this program, you need to take two scoops of protein powder that has around 50 grams of protein and 2 to 4 capsules of multivitamins after the meal. If you are on any medication, please consult your doctor before taking these capsules.

CALORIES

C alories have two units: calories (Cal) and kilocalories (Kcal). Don't get confused between these two. If you think that it has the word "kilo" in it, which means 1000 calories = 1 kilocalorie, then you are incorrect. Both units have the same meaning. 300 calories and 300 kilocalories are one and the same.

While I told you to eat vegetables, fruits, grains, nuts, etc., I am not going to tell you how much of each you need to eat. It is perfectly fine to eat spinach in the vegetable category, apple or banana in the fruit category, a bowl of rice in the grain category, walnut, almond, or cashew in the nut category, and chicken, soya or fish in the protein category. What this program needs from you is to count your calories. Whatever you eat, you have to calculate your calories. Some of you might say counting calories is a very tedious job, but don't worry, I am going to make it very simple for you.

Different food items will be available in different regions according to the season. But if you look closely at your daily food intake, you will find that there are some common foods that you eat regularly on a daily basis. The same common food is found in our mills 70% of the time. And while these common foods are few, you can count them on your fingers. So you have to make a list of those common foods and you have to write down their calories for a hundred grams or one-count.

For instance, if you have an egg in your common food, then add it to this list.

1 whole egg - 78 Cal

The next step in this program is to determine how many calories you must eat each day. Suppose you have to consume 1600 calories on a particular day and you've included 3 whole eggs in your diet plan for that day. Therefore, you will consume 78x3=234 calories from the egg and the remaining calories from some other foods.

In this program, there will be calorie changes only five times in 30 days. You would start with 2400 calories, which would come down to 800 calories in the following sequence.

2400 calories
2000 calories
1600 calories
1200 calories
800 calories

So before starting the program, you have to prepare your diet plan, which will be divided into 5 parts. We will try to consume a healthy diet during these 30 days. Make a list of the foods you want to have in the next 30 days. Put some variety in that list as well. Suppose you have to consume 1600 calories for 5 days. If you eat 3 eggs every day for those 5 days, then you will probably get bored. So, if you can exchange 234 calories from 3 eggs for another food, such as sprouts, you will have more variety in your diet and you will enjoy it more. Remember that you just have to pay attention to how many calories are in these foods. Pay no attention to the amount of protein, carbohydrates, or fat in 1 egg. Pay attention only to calories.

WEIGHING MACHINE

W hen you stand on the weighing machine every day or every alternate day, and if you see that you have lost a few pounds, then you will get very excited. You will be motivated to do those things which got you this result. The opposite is equally true. If your weight on the weighing machine shows the same digits, appears higher than before or does not show according to your expectations, then you become disappointed and you do not get the motivation to do more work. And we can't afford to be demotivated in this program. This program has therefore established a strict rule regarding when to check your weight. For the first time, you have to measure your weight the day before starting the program. And after that, you have to measure your weight only 3 times during the entire program and that will be on the 11th day, the 20th day, and the last 30th day.

Always check your weight in the morning when you come back from exercise. You will get the best digits on the machine this time because it is the final phase of intermittent fasting and you will have burned off the extra calories from running and skipping. You must strictly adhere to the rule of checking your weight, because I don't want you to get discouraged in the middle of the journey. This journey is very short, so don't pay too much attention to the result in between. Just follow the process and you will see that the end results will mesmerize you completely.

VACATION

Most of you get a weekly day off on Saturdays and Sundays, but you will not get any leave in this 30-Day Guided Weight Loss Program. Every day you have to do all three elements of this program which are exercise, diet, and intermittent fasting. The rest that your body needs will be available only when you sleep at night.

In the next 30 days, be a bit selfish and focus solely on yourself and your body. Make this program your priority and be extremely devoted to it. Do not take even a single day off or break in the coming 30 days. Therefore, whenever you plan to follow this program, just check if any important work is coming up in the next 30 days that requires your attention and you need to go out of town for some days. If that is the case, try not to start the program. Go finish your important work, and then you can start the program straight for 30 days without any interruptions.

Having said that, sometimes there will be circumstances that we cannot avoid. For example, you may fall sick or a family emergency may come and it needs your absolute attention and you cannot continue the program. In such circumstances, we can adjust the program a bit.

Suppose, after following the program for 15 days, you need to take a gap of 3 days, so after the gap, you must resume the program in the following manner.

The program is completed until the 15th day

(15th day) - (3 day gap) = 12th day.

You have to resume the program on the 12th day. So, whatever diet and exercise you did on the 12th day, you must do the same on the first day after the break. Then, you can continue with the regular program for 30 days. So if there is a gap, just subtract the number of gap days from the particular day of the program where you left and then just continue.

If the emergency gap happens after only 5 days of starting the program, then I would recommend starting the program from day 1. If the emergency gap comes on the 25th day, you are still required to continue the last 5 days after the gap. The program must be followed for the entire 30 days.

So we can adjust the program a bit in emergency situations, but I would like to see you follow the program continuously without interruption.

GYM

Many of my clients were those who were already enrolled in gym memberships and, despite going to the gym, they were not getting the results they wanted. Whenever they approached me about this program, their first question would always be, "Can I do this in the gym?" My answer would always be, "No."

I used to tell them that I wanted to take them out of the gym to a different environment. I want you to do this program under the open sky with nature. And for this, you will have to take a gap of 1 month from your gym. This program will help you reduce your weight and body fat percentage if you are overweight. Then you can join the gym and do weight training to shape your body. It also depends on what your goal is. The goal of most of my clients was to get rid of their obesity in some way, and when they achieved it, they started following a healthy lifestyle every day to maintain their fitness. A healthy lifestyle means they used to exercise 4 to 5 times a week, which included running, skipping, sit-ups, pull-ups, and push-ups. Plus, they did intermittent fasting and ate a healthy diet.

The goal of some clients was to achieve a desirable body shape. I used to advise them to join a gym as soon as they lost weight by following a 30-day weight loss program. Rather than going to the gym and doing weight training, if you are overweight, I suggest you work on that extra fat first and then do weight training.

I knew a gym member whose hands and legs were thin but had a big belly. And he loved doing all the abs exercises. He thought that if he worked on his abs, his belly fat would be reduced. He used to work hard on his abs, but he did not like doing cardio in the gym at all. He once showed me his fat belly in the changing room. He took a deep breath and pulled his stomach in. I saw that his abs muscles had taken a very good shape behind the fat layer of his stomach. But due to the upper layer of fat, abs were not visible to anyone. He released his breath and his belly popped out. He then asked me what to do with this balloon. I said, "Run."

HUNGER

Intermittent fasting is a very important part of our program. Since fasting is in its name, you have to stay away from food most of the time. As we progress in the program, the period of fasting will increase gradually. In such a situation, it is expected to feel hungry. So what do you do when you feel hungry? There are some remedies for this problem too.

All the volunteers in the spiritual leader Sadhguru's Isha foundation get food only twice a day; the first meal is served at 10 a.m. in the morning and the second at 7 p.m. in the evening. Usually, his volunteers feel very hungry around 5 p.m. He says to them that no matter how much you hold your stomach and say, "Sadhguru, we are feeling very hungry," you will only get the food at the appointed time. By the way, let me tell you that Sadhguru himself takes only 1 meal a day.

1] Zero-Calorie Beverages:

You can drink some beverages like black coffee, green tea, or black tea during your fasting window. These beverages will reduce your appetite a bit, and you will feel relieved. Keep in mind that zero calories should be written in front of calories in the nutritional facts of whatever beverage you are consuming. In general, all these beverages do not contain calories, but some brands have extra calories because of added flavors. So, before you drink your favorite beverage, remember to check the calories. If we want zero calories, then it is obvious that we do not have to add any extras to them, such as milk, sugar, cream, etc. Your location will also have some zero-calorie drinks or beverages besides coffee and tea. You can also include that in your fasting window.

2] Water:

The duration of the fasting window is longer and we can't have black coffee or green tea all the time. That is why, whenever my clients used to be hungry, they used to drink the healthiest drink in the world, which is water. You will not find a better drink than water. Always keep a water bottle at the place where you work, and whenever you feel a bit hungry, have water; you will feel a lot relieved.

3] Vipassana:

Vipassana is an ancient yoga science in India. It is a Buddhist term. We can use this ancient yoga to solve our hunger. In Vipassana Yoga, you are taught that any sensation arising in your body is not permanent. If the sensation has arisen, then it will also go away. Hunger is also a sensation that arises in our stomach, and this sensation is also mortal. It is temporary. It will come and go. So how can we use Vipassana Yoga in our program?

Whenever you feel hungry, close your eyes and pay attention to where you are feeling the sensation of hunger in your stomach. Sometimes it is on the right side of the stomach and sometimes on the left; sometimes above, sometimes below; sometimes in the middle part of the stomach. Pay close attention wherever there is a feeling of hunger. Sometimes the sensation will be mild and sometimes it will be intense. Experience the sensation as it is. There is a feeling of hunger, and it is true, and that is why you should not ignore it. Pay more attention to it. You will find that the intensity of hunger will gradually decrease. All the sensations are all mortal. Sensation of hunger is there, but only for a while. It's temporary, not permanent. It will go. If you pay close attention to the sensation, then it will end and you will not feel hungry anymore. This is the magic of yoga.

LISTEN TO YOUR BODY

In this 30-day time period, we will push our physical capacity a bit. There will be many of you who have never run more than 2 miles. Many people have never considered running as an exercise. All of you have to push your physical boundaries. Day by day, this program will present new challenges to you for the next 30 days. And you have to overcome all the challenges daily. As the program progresses, your challenges and difficulties will increase. The distance of running and the quantity of skipping will increase. The fasting window will be longer, and the calories will be fewer. All this will happen within 30 days, and your body is so capable that it can easily withstand even more difficult situations.

There are some yogis in India who have surprised even medical science with their physical abilities. There is a yogi in India who, after turning 40, remains alive only by taking sunlight. He neither eats nor drinks water. He died when he was 90 years old. He lived without water and food for 50 years.

Some yogis sit naked and meditate in the snow of

the Himalayas. And even at -10 to -30 degree Celsius, they survive for many days. The purpose of telling you all this is to show that the capability of your body is endless. Your body is capable of doing many more challenges than what you have been given in this program. I have named this topic "Listen to your body," because even though our body's ability is amazing, sometimes our body gives us some signs to which we should pay attention.

If today's challenge is to run 6 miles, and after running constantly for 3 miles, your heartbeat becomes very fast, then you have to stop at that point. You can complete the last 3 miles after taking some rest. The objective of this program is to run 6 miles, not 6 miles nonstop.

Everything depends on you. You can run fast, slow, or intermittently in between. If your body is supporting you very well as you run continuously for 3 miles but your mind tells you to stop, there is no need to listen to your mind. At that time, you can motivate yourself to run an extra 1 mile and complete 4 miles in one go. Your mind wants to give you comfort most of the time, and if you always listen to your mind, it will be very difficult to make changes in your body. So, listen to your body but don't listen to your mind always.

You must ensure that you are completely fit before beginning the program. Aside from obesity, you should not have any health problems. Because we will push the limits of our bodies in this program, being healthy is crucial. If you are currently taking any medications, you should consult your doctor before starting this program.

Let's say today is Day-17 and your challenge is to run for 4 miles and do 340 skips. Suppose after running for 2 miles, your ankle gets twisted, you get cramps, or you feel dizzy, and you cannot continue the rest of the challenge. What should you do then?

Simply return home and write the following on the page of Day-17.

I ran 2 miles today. I will add the remaining 2 miles and 340 skips of today's challenge in the coming day or two.

If you leave these remaining miles and skips, then your mind will find an excuse to postpone another day's challenge as well. But if you are dedicated to completing it in the next day or two, then you are not giving your mind any chance to find an excuse. Add 1 mile and 170 skips on Day-18 and rest on Day-19. Do not exceed more than 2 days because the coming challenges will be much more difficult to complete. It will be tough to add more to that.

If you are fasting for 20 hours and taking 1200 calories on Day 17, and if you feel recurring dizziness, then you need to have electrolyte powder or some energy drink. It is not recommended that you compensate for today's missed intermittent fasting the next day.

PLANNING
VS DOING

No matter how good the plan is, it is useless until you start working on it. The weight you have gained has not increased in one day. Many burgers, pizzas, snacks, and delicious dishes have made their contribution to your current weight. For many years, you ate continuously, had a late-night dinner, and in a few cases, even a beer belly would have come out. Ask a thin person whose weight doesn't increase despite all the efforts. He will ask you, "How did you manage to put on weight?" I am trying, but it's not happening with me. I bet you must have worked hard for many years to gain weight."

The hard work you put in for so many years unknowingly gave you this result of being overweight, and it's not a pleasant result. So, if you want to return to your previous self, you must work much harder.

It is common for people to take a few steps on their way to losing weight, but then give up after seeing no results. Whatever you say, the human mind works in such a way that it likes to see the result. Only 5% people continue to work hard even though they don't see any results. And because they are persistent, one day they get the results. If you were counting yourself among those 5%, then it would be a big mistake, because if that were the case, then you would not need this book. Sorry, but it's true. And there is nothing to feel bad about that because, at the end of the day, the result matters. We have to make our bodies fit. That is our mission, and we are going to work hard for that.

Someone once said, "To gain something, you have to lose something." And to succeed in this program, you have to lose procrastination, hunger, and all the negative things that can become obstacles in your way of achieving what you want. You have to remain fully charged for the next 30 days. You should not let any negative thoughts wander around. Watch at least 2 motivational videos every day for the next 30 days. One video before going to sleep and another after you wake up. Apart from this, whenever a negative thought surrounds you, you start watching inspirational videos. You just have to keep in mind that whatever hard work you do, it is only for 30 days. I will tell you in the next chapter what you have to do exactly after 30 days. But for now, you just have to think about the next 30 days.

You have to think of a big reward for yourself. That reward can be anything of your choice. For someone, that reward would be a favorite holiday destination. For someone, that would be some materialistic thing that they could gift to themselves. That reward can be anything you like very much. The reward is for achieving the best results by working hard every day for these 30 days. Enjoy it wholeheartedly, because you deserve it.

WHAT TO DO AFTER FINISHING THIS PROGRAM?

If you have followed this program regularly every day for 30 days, then you will definitely get the result, because it is a tried and tested method. One of my clients, Mrs. Poonam Bhatia, was 74 pounds away from her ideal weight when she started this program. She lost 26 pounds in 30 days. She was very happy and very motivated, and she asked me what she should do to reduce another 48 pounds.

After 30 days of completion, I generally do not keep my clients' programs very rigorous. I tell them to take 2 meals a day during the eating window of intermittent fasting and follow a healthy diet. Run for about 4 to 5 miles and do 200 to 300 skips. What it will do is it will slow down the weight-reducing intensity a little bit. But don't get disappointed because the plus point is that you are still continuously reducing your weight and you can follow this till your ideal weight is achieved.

Now, I am not going to spoon-feed you. The miles

to run and the numbers to skip are not fixed. After finishing this 30-day weight loss program, you will know exactly how your body reacts to exercise and dieting. On that basis, you have to plan for yourself what exactly you want to do. You can write your own plan for the next 30 days because you now know how the weight loss program works. Now you have to decide how much running, skipping, intermittent fasting, and dieting you have to do. But when you are doing this, you have to sit down and do proper planning with a pen and paper in your hand or on your laptop. Write down how you intend to proceed with your weight loss plan over the next 30 days.

Again, listen to your body. One of my clients followed the 30th day program for the next 2 months, and the results were mesmerizing. He listened to his body. His body, mind, and energy allowed him to continue the program. So after 30 days, it's your call on what to do. But whatever you do, don't get back to what you were doing before.

There may come a point in your weight loss process where after reaching a particular weight, your weight has become stuck and it is even difficult to reduce a pound or 2. This is called a stagnant state. This state also occurs in those who want to gain weight. In this state, you need to put in the extra effort. A further 2 miles of running, hundreds more skips, intermittent fasting with just 1 meal each day, and so forth. You have to push yourself harder to get out of that stagnant state.

You will enjoy listening to the daily rituals of many of my clients who have achieved ideal weight. They run daily for around 3 miles and do 100 to 200 skips. Some clients include pull-ups, push-ups, and sit-ups in their workouts. And to do all this, they give only 30 to 40 minutes and they mostly follow intermittent fasting. They do not follow it rigorously. If they are at a party or on a trip, then they skip it. They have now adopted a healthy lifestyle. This does not mean that they have stopped eating pizza and burgers. They do enjoy all the food, but also take care of their bodies. If your ideal weight is 130 pounds, then maintain your weight at around 125 to 129 pounds. If it increases to 131 pounds, then follow intermittent fasting very strictly for a few days. The most important thing is that, after achieving their ideal weight, my clients are now enjoying their new fit life. And I want you to reach this point as soon as possible.

30-DAY GUIDED WEIGHT LOSS PROGRAM

How to use this book?

Before going to bed every night, prepare yourself for the next day. Keep your running shoes and jumping rope handy. If you carry a waist pouch or a backpack, then pack all the items you require for your running and skipping in it, like water bottle, hand towel, mobile phone, jumping rope, etc.

If the number of calories and meals change the next day, you must prepare for the diet the day before. Buy all the food items in advance that you will require for the next day's diet. Just be totally prepared.

At night, read tomorrow's challenge and prepare yourself mentally for it. Watch motivational videos of running and skipping before going to bed and after waking up. Please look at the format of the daily challenge page below.

DATE- _____

    ☐   I have completed my running challenge

for today.

☐   I have completed my skipping challenge for today.

☐   I have followed my diet and intermittent fasting for today.

Once you have completed the challenge for today, enter the date and check the first 2 boxes. After your last meal, check the last box if you've followed the diet and intermittent fasting for the day.

Rajat, what if I could only complete 70% of the challenge in a day?

First of all, don't do that. I mean, this program is for your own benefit and you have to follow it for only 30 days. Make your mind so strong for the next 30 days that no force in this world can stop you. Even if it's raining, snow falling, or windy outside, it doesn't matter, just go for a run and jump the rope. Don't look for excuses. If you search, you will easily find an excuse not to complete the task. If today's task is to complete running for 3 miles and 450 skips and there is a storm and lightning outside, then run on the treadmill. Oh, but I don't have a treadmill. That's so expensive. That is another excuse. I told you that finding an excuse would be simple. If you don't have a treadmill, then just do skips, but not 450; do 1000 skips to compensate for the running. My legs will hurt if I do that many skips. That is another excuse. Who told you to do all 1000 skips on the go? Take a break as much as you can. You can put on some music and do aerobics for 20 minutes.

You can do push-ups, sit-ups, and all the bodyweight exercises and burn some calories to compensate for the running that you couldn't do because of the extreme weather conditions. Whatever the reason, finish the day's challenge. Just do it.

As far as intermittent fasting is concerned, the only problem you will face is hunger. And I already told you some tricks on how to cope with hunger in chapter 12. Guys, it's a matter of 30 days. Just give it your all. Because the result you will see on the 30th day will mesmerize you. It will give you so much energy and confidence in your life that you will never regret putting in the effort for these 30 days.

For the next 30 days, pick a book you have already read that inspires you and read it daily. Make a playlist of all the inspirational videos on YouTube and keep on watching them throughout this program. You can listen to some inspirational podcasts. Just keep yourself motivated day in and out for the next 30 days. If you stick to the program for 30 days, then the results are very fruitful. You will be amazed by your body and mind's capacity to achieve success in life. Are you ready? Let's begin the "30-Day Guided Weight Loss Program."

DAY 1

RUNNING
Depart (D) - 0.5 Miles
Arrive (A) - 0.5 Miles
Total Running = 1 Mile

SKIPPING - 20 Skips

DIETING - 3 MEALS - 2400 Calories

INTERMITTENT FASTING
Fasting Window - 16 hours
Eating Window - 8 hours

WEIGHT - _____ Pounds

DATE - _____

- ☐ I have completed my running challenge for today.
- ☐ I have completed my skipping challenge for today.
- ☐ I have followed my diet and intermittent fasting for today.

I have started the 30 day weight loss program pretty well. I am feeling great and have endless energy. I am mentally and physically ready for my 2nd day challenge. Let's lose this damn weight faster.

DAY 2

RUNNING
Depart (D) - 0.55 Miles
Arrive (A) - 0.55 Miles
Total Running = 1.1 Miles

SKIPPING - 40 Skips

DIETING - 3 MEALS - 2400 Calories

INTERMITTENT FASTING
Fasting Window - 16 hours
Eating Window - 8 hours

DATE - _____

- ☐ I have completed my running challenge for today.
- ☐ I have completed my skipping challenge for today.
- ☐ I have followed my diet and intermittent fasting for today.

I am feeling great and have endless energy. I am mentally and physically ready for my 3rd day challenge. Let's lose this damn weight faster.

DAY 3

RUNNING
Depart (D) - 0.6 Miles
Arrive (A) - 0.6 Miles
Total Running = 1.2 Miles

SKIPPING - 60 Skips

DIETING - 3 MEALS - 2400 Calories

INTERMITTENT FASTING
Fasting Window - 16 hours
Eating Window - 8 hours

DATE - _____

- ☐ I have completed my running challenge for today.
- ☐ I have completed my skipping challenge for today.
- ☐ I have followed my diet and intermittent fasting for today.

I am feeling great and have endless energy. I am mentally and physically ready for my 4th day challenge. Let's lose this damn weight faster.

DAY 4

RUNNING
Depart (D) - 0.65 Miles
Arrive (A) - 0.65 Miles
Total Running = 1.3 Miles

SKIPPING - 80 Skips

DIETING - 3 MEALS - 2400 Calories

INTERMITTENT FASTING
Fasting Window - 16 hours
Eating Window - 8 hours

DATE - _____

- ☐   I have completed my running challenge for today.
- ☐   I have completed my skipping challenge for today.
- ☐   I have followed my diet and intermittent fasting for today.

I am feeling great and have endless energy. I am mentally and physically ready for my 5th day challenge. Let's lose this damn weight faster.

DAY 5

RUNNING
Depart (D) - 0.7 Miles
Arrive (A) - 0.7 Miles
Total Running = 1.4 Miles

SKIPPING - 100 Skips

DIETING - 3 MEALS - 2400 Calories

INTERMITTENT FASTING
Fasting Window - 16 hours
Eating Window - 8 hours

DATE - _____

- ☐   I have completed my running challenge for today.
- ☐   I have completed my skipping challenge for today.
- ☐   I have followed my diet and intermittent fasting for today.

I am feeling great and have endless energy. I am mentally and physically ready for my 6th day challenge. Let's lose this damn weight faster.

DAY 6

RUNNING
Depart (D) - 0.75 Miles
Arrive (A) - 0.75 Miles
Total Running = 1.5 Miles

SKIPPING - 120 Skips

DIETING - 3 MEALS - 2000 Calories

INTERMITTENT FASTING
Fasting Window - 16 hours
Eating Window - 8 hours

DATE - _____

- ☐   I have completed my running challenge for today.
- ☐   I have completed my skipping challenge for today.
- ☐   I have followed my diet and intermittent fasting for today.

I am feeling great and have endless energy. I am mentally and physically ready for my 7th day challenge. Let's lose this damn weight faster.

DAY 7

RUNNING
Depart (D) - 0.85 Miles
Arrive (A) - 0.85 Miles
Total Running = 1.7 Miles

SKIPPING - 140 Skips

DIETING - 3 MEALS - 2000 Calories

INTERMITTENT FASTING
Fasting Window - 16 hours
Eating Window - 8 hours

DATE - _____

- ☐ I have completed my running challenge for today.
- ☐ I have completed my skipping challenge for today.
- ☐ I have followed my diet and intermittent fasting for today.

I am feeling great and have endless energy. I am mentally and physically ready for my 8th day challenge. Let's lose this damn weight faster.

DAY 8

RUNNING
Depart (D) - 0.95 Miles
Arrive (A) - 0.95 Miles
Total Running = 1.9 Miles

SKIPPING - 160 Skips

DIETING - 3 MEALS - 2000 Calories

INTERMITTENT FASTING
Fasting Window - 16 hours
Eating Window - 8 hours

DATE - _____

- ☐   I have completed my running challenge for today.
- ☐   I have completed my skipping challenge for today.
- ☐   I have followed my diet and intermittent fasting for today.

I am feeling great and have endless energy. I am mentally and physically ready for my 9th day challenge. Let's lose this damn weight faster.

DAY 9

RUNNING
Depart (D) - 1.05 Miles
Arrive (A) - 1.05 Miles
Total Running = 2.1 Miles

SKIPPING - 180 Skips

DIETING - 3 MEALS - 2000 Calories

INTERMITTENT FASTING
Fasting Window - 16 hours
Eating Window - 8 hours

DATE - _____

☐   I have completed my running challenge for today.
☐   I have completed my skipping challenge for today.
☐   I have followed my diet and intermittent fasting for today.

I am feeling great and have endless energy. I am mentally and physically ready for my 10th day challenge. Let's lose this damn weight faster.

DAY 10

RUNNING
Depart (D) - 1.15 Miles
Arrive (A) - 1.15 Miles
Total Running = 2.3 Miles

SKIPPING - 200 Skips

DIETING - 3 MEALS - 2000 Calories

INTERMITTENT FASTING
Fasting Window - 16 hours
Eating Window - 8 hours

DATE - _____

- ☐   I have completed my running challenge for today.
- ☐   I have completed my skipping challenge for today.
- ☐   I have followed my diet and intermittent fasting for today.

I am feeling great and have endless energy. I am mentally and physically ready for my 11th day challenge. Let's lose this damn weight faster.

DAY 11

RUNNING
Depart (D) - 1.25 Miles
Arrive (A) - 1.25 Miles
Total Running = 2.5 Miles

SKIPPING - 220 Skips

DIETING - 2 MEALS - 1600 Calories

INTERMITTENT FASTING
Fasting Window - 18 hours
Eating Window - 6 hours

WEIGHT - _____Pounds

DATE - _____

- ☐ I have completed my running challenge for today.
- ☐ I have completed my skipping challenge for today.
- ☐ I have followed my diet and intermittent fasting for today.

I am feeling great and have endless energy. I am mentally and physically ready for my 12th day challenge. Let's lose this damn weight faster.

DAY 12

RUNNING
Depart (D) - 1.35 Miles
Arrive (A) - 1.35 Miles
Total Running = 2.7 Miles

SKIPPING - 240 Skips

DIETING - 2 MEALS - 1600 Calories

INTERMITTENT FASTING
Fasting Window - 18 hours
Eating Window - 6 hours

DATE - _____

- ☐ I have completed my running challenge for today.
- ☐ I have completed my skipping challenge for today.
- ☐ I have followed my diet and intermittent fasting for today.

I am feeling great and have endless energy. I am mentally and physically ready for my 13th day challenge. Let's lose this damn weight faster.

DAY 13

RUNNING
Depart (D) - 1.45 Miles
Arrive (A) - 1.45 Miles
Total Running = 2.9 Miles

SKIPPING - 260 Skips

DIETING - 2 MEALS - 1600 Calories

INTERMITTENT FASTING
Fasting Window - 18 hours
Eating Window - 6 hours

DATE - _____

- ☐ I have completed my running challenge for today.
- ☐ I have completed my skipping challenge for today.
- ☐ I have followed my diet and intermittent fasting for today.

I am feeling great and have endless energy. I am mentally and physically ready for my 14th day challenge. Let's lose this damn weight faster.

DAY 14

RUNNING
Depart (D) - 1.55 Miles
Arrive (A) - 1.55 Miles
Total Running = 3.1 Miles

SKIPPING - 280 Skips

DIETING - 2 MEALS - 1600 Calories

INTERMITTENT FASTING
Fasting Window - 18 hours
Eating Window - 6 hours

DATE - _____

- ☐ I have completed my running challenge for today.
- ☐ I have completed my skipping challenge for today.
- ☐ I have followed my diet and intermittent fasting for today.

I am feeling great and have endless energy. I am mentally and physically ready for my 15th day challenge. Let's lose this damn weight faster.

DAY 15

RUNNING
Depart (D) - 1.7 Miles
Arrive (A) - 1.7 Miles
Total Running = 3.4 Miles

SKIPPING - 300 Skips

DIETING - 2 MEALS - 1600 Calories

INTERMITTENT FASTING
Fasting Window - 18 hours
Eating Window - 6 hours

DATE - _____

- ☐ I have completed my running challenge for today.
- ☐ I have completed my skipping challenge for today.
- ☐ I have followed my diet and intermittent fasting for today.

I am feeling great and have endless energy. I am mentally and physically ready for my 16th day challenge. Let's lose this damn weight faster.

DAY 16

RUNNING
Depart (D) - 1.85 Miles
Arrive (A) - 1.85 Miles
Total Running = 3.7 Miles

SKIPPING - 320 Skips

DIETING - 2 MEALS - 1600 Calories

INTERMITTENT FASTING
Fasting Window - 18 hours
Eating Window - 6 hours

DATE - _____

- ☐   I have completed my running challenge for today.
- ☐   I have completed my skipping challenge for today.
- ☐   I have followed my diet and intermittent fasting for today.

I am feeling great and have endless energy. I am mentally and physically ready for my 17th day challenge. Let's lose this damn weight faster.

DAY 17

RUNNING
Depart (D) - 2 Miles
Arrive (A) - 2 Miles
Total Running = 4 Miles

SKIPPING - 340 Skips

DIETING - 2 MEALS - 1200 Calories

INTERMITTENT FASTING
Fasting Window - 20 hours
Eating Window - 4 hours

DATE - _____

- ☐ I have completed my running challenge for today.
- ☐ I have completed my skipping challenge for today.
- ☐   I have followed my diet and intermittent fasting for today.

I am feeling great and have endless energy. I am mentally and physically ready for my 18th day challenge. Let's lose this damn weight faster.

DAY 18

RUNNING
Depart (D) - 2.15 Miles
Arrive (A) - 2.15 Miles
Total Running = 4.3 Miles

SKIPPING - 360 Skips

DIETING - 2 MEALS - 1200 Calories

INTERMITTENT FASTING
Fasting Window - 20 hours
Eating Window - 4 hours

DATE - _____

- ☐ I have completed my running challenge for today.
- ☐ I have completed my skipping challenge for today.
- ☐ I have followed my diet and intermittent fasting for today.

I am feeling great and have endless energy. I am mentally and physically ready for my 19th day challenge. Let's lose this damn weight faster.

DAY 19

RUNNING
Depart (D) - 2.3 Miles
Arrive (A) - 2.3 Miles
Total Running = 4.6 Miles

SKIPPING - 380 Skips

DIETING - 2 MEALS - 1200 Calories

INTERMITTENT FASTING
Fasting Window - 20 hours
Eating Window - 4 hours

DATE - _____

- ☐   I have completed my running challenge for today.
- ☐   I have completed my skipping challenge for today.
- ☐   I have followed my diet and intermittent fasting for today.

I am feeling great and have endless energy. I am mentally and physically ready for my 20th day challenge. Let's lose this damn weight faster.

DAY 20

RUNNING
Depart (D) - 2.5 Miles
Arrive (A) - 2.5 Miles
Total Running = 5 Miles

SKIPPING - 400 Skips

DIETING - 2 MEALS - 1200 Calories

INTERMITTENT FASTING
Fasting Window - 20 hours
Eating Window - 4 hours

WEIGHT - _____Pounds

DATE - _____

- ☐ I have completed my running challenge for today.
- ☐ I have completed my skipping challenge for today.
- ☐ I have followed my diet and intermittent fasting for today.

I am feeling great and have endless energy. I am mentally and physically ready for my 21st day challenge. Let's lose this damn weight faster.

DAY 21

RUNNING
Depart (D) - 2.7 Miles
Arrive (A) - 2.7 Miles
Total Running = 5.4 Miles

SKIPPING - 420 Skips

DIETING - 1 MEAL - 1200 Calories

INTERMITTENT FASTING
Fasting Window - 23 hours
Eating Window - 1 hours

DATE - _____

- ☐ I have completed my running challenge for today.
- ☐ I have completed my skipping challenge for today.
- ☐ I have followed my diet and intermittent fasting for today.

I am feeling great and have endless energy. I am mentally and physically ready for my 22nd day challenge. Let's lose this damn weight faster.

DAY 22

RUNNING
Depart (D) - 2.9 Miles
Arrive (A) - 2.9 Miles
Total Running = 5.8 Miles

SKIPPING - 440 Skips

DIETING - 1 MEAL - 1200 Calories

INTERMITTENT FASTING
Fasting Window - 23 hours
Eating Window - 1 hours

DATE - _____

- ☐ I have completed my running challenge for today.
- ☐ I have completed my skipping challenge for today.
- ☐ I have followed my diet and intermittent fasting for today.

I am feeling great and have endless energy. I am mentally and physically ready for my 23rd day challenge. Let's lose this damn weight faster.

DAY 23

RUNNING
Depart (D) - 3.1 Miles
Arrive (A) - 3.1 Miles
Total Running = 6.2 Miles

SKIPPING - 460 Skips

DIETING - 1 MEAL - 1200 Calories

INTERMITTENT FASTING
Fasting Window - 23 hours
Eating Window - 1 hours

DATE - _____

- ☐ I have completed my running challenge for today.
- ☐ I have completed my skipping challenge for today.
- ☐ I have followed my diet and intermittent fasting for today.

I am feeling great and have endless energy. I am mentally and physically ready for my 24th day challenge. Let's lose this damn weight faster.

DAY 24

RUNNING
Depart (D) - 3.35 Miles
Arrive (A) - 3.35 Miles
Total Running = 6.7 Miles

SKIPPING - 480 Skips

DIETING - 1 MEAL - 800 Calories

INTERMITTENT FASTING
Fasting Window - 23 hours
Eating Window - 1 hours

DATE - _____

- ☐ I have completed my running challenge for today.
- ☐ I have completed my skipping challenge for today.
- ☐ I have followed my diet and intermittent fasting for today.

I am feeling great and have endless energy. I am mentally and physically ready for my 25th day challenge. Let's lose this damn weight faster.

DAY 25

RUNNING
Depart (D) - 3.6 Miles
Arrive (A) - 3.6 Miles
Total Running = 7.2 Miles

SKIPPING - 500 Skips

DIETING - 1 MEAL - 800 Calories

INTERMITTENT FASTING
Fasting Window - 23 hours
Eating Window - 1 hours

DATE - _____

- ☐ I have completed my running challenge for today.
- ☐ I have completed my skipping challenge for today.
- ☐ I have followed my diet and intermittent fasting for today.

I am feeling great and have endless energy. I am mentally and physically ready for my 26th day challenge. Let's lose this damn weight faster.

DAY 26

RUNNING
Depart (D) - 3.85 Miles
Arrive (A) - 3.85 Miles
Total Running = 7.7 Miles

SKIPPING - 520 Skips

DIETING - 1 MEAL - 800 Calories

INTERMITTENT FASTING
Fasting Window - 23 hours
Eating Window - 1 hours

DATE - _____

- ☐ I have completed my running challenge for today.
- ☐ I have completed my skipping challenge for today.
- ☐ I have followed my diet and intermittent fasting for today.

I am feeling great and have endless energy. I am mentally and physically ready for my 27th day challenge. Let's lose this damn weight faster.

DAY 27

RUNNING
Depart (D) - 4.1 Miles
Arrive (A) - 4.1 Miles
Total Running = 8.2 Miles

SKIPPING - 540 Skips

DIETING - 1 MEAL - 800 Calories

INTERMITTENT FASTING
Fasting Window - 23 hours
Eating Window - 1 hours

DATE - _____

- ☐ I have completed my running challenge for today.
- ☐ I have completed my skipping challenge for today.
- ☐ I have followed my diet and intermittent fasting for today.

I am feeling great and have endless energy. I am mentally and physically ready for my 28th day challenge. Let's lose this damn weight faster.

DAY 28

RUNNING
Depart (D) - 4.4 Miles
Arrive (A) - 4.4 Miles
Total Running = 8.8 Miles

SKIPPING - 560 Skips

DIETING - 1 MEAL - 800 Calories

INTERMITTENT FASTING
Fasting Window - 23 hours
Eating Window - 1 hours

DATE - _____

- ☐   I have completed my running challenge for today.
- ☐   I have completed my skipping challenge for today.
- ☐   I have followed my diet and intermittent fasting for today.

I am feeling great and have endless energy. I am mentally and physically ready for my 29th day challenge. Let's lose this damn weight faster.

DAY 29

RUNNING
Depart (D) - 4.7 Miles
Arrive (A) - 4.7 Miles
Total Running = 9.4 Miles

SKIPPING - 580 Skips

DIETING - 1 MEAL - 800 Calories

INTERMITTENT FASTING
Fasting Window - 23 hours
Eating Window - 1 hours

DATE - _____

- ☐ I have completed my running challenge for today.
- ☐ I have completed my skipping challenge for today.
- ☐ I have followed my diet and intermittent fasting for today.

I am feeling great and have endless energy. I am mentally and physically ready for my 30th day challenge. Let's lose this damn weight faster.

DAY 30

RUNNING
Depart (D) - 5 Miles
Arrive (A) - 5 Miles
Total Running = 10 Miles

SKIPPING - 600 Skips

DIETING - 1 MEAL - 800 Calories

INTERMITTENT FASTING
Fasting Window - 23 hours
Eating Window - 1 hours

WEIGHT - _____Pounds

DATE - _____

- ☐ I have completed my running challenge for today.
- ☐ I have completed my skipping challenge for today.
- ☐ I have followed my diet and intermittent fasting for today.

I am feeling great and have endless energy. I have successfully completed my 30-Day Weight Loss Program. When I started the program my weight was _____ pounds. I have lost _____ pounds in the last 30 days. My current weight is _____pounds. This is the best result I have ever achieved in my attempt to lose weight. I am going to follow a healthy lifestyle from now onwards. Because I have come to know that health is everything.

CONCLUSION

Guys, many years pass by in our lives without us even realizing it. Years fly by so quickly, forget about months, and you have to take only one month out of those many months. Only 30 days. If you give your full dedication to this program, you will see results that will blow your mind.

Now is the time to start caring for your body. If you pay attention to your body, your body will pay attention to you. Go ahead and prepare vigorously for the next 30 days.

Last but not least, I would like to see your 30-day transformation. Please upload your before and after 30-day photos to the Amazon review. I would also like to see photos of the weighing scale before and after 30 days. I'd be delighted to witness your transformation. If you have questions about the program, feel free to ask me.

Email id - rajatbgajbhiye@gmail.com.

Work Hard. All the best.

Printed in Great Britain
by Amazon